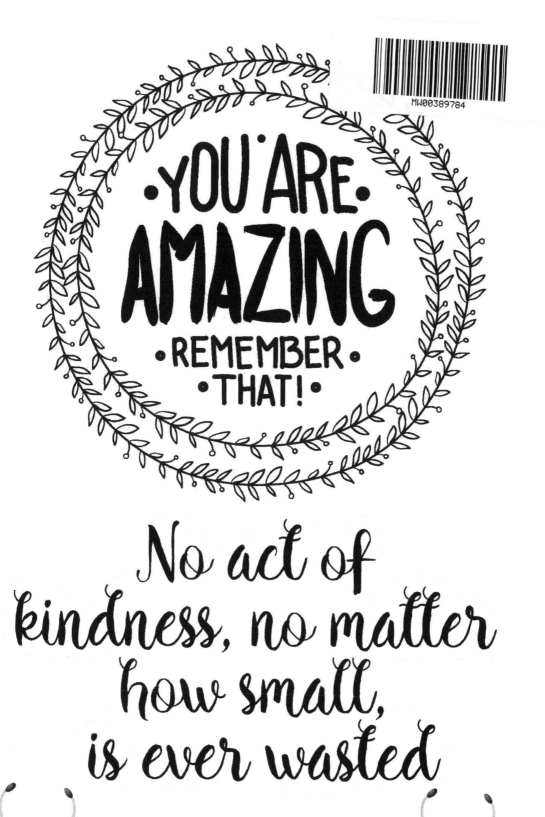

·YOU·ARE·
AMAZING
·REMEMBER·
·THAT!·

No act of
kindness, no matter
how small,
is ever wasted

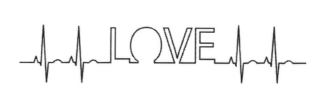

Nurse Life

○ MONDAY

PRIORITIES

○ TUESDAY

○ WEDNESDAY

TO DO

○ THURSDAY

○ FRIDAY

○ SATURDAY / SUNDAY

MEALS / FOOD

MISCELLANEOUS

ME TIME - READ, WALK, RELAX, SPA, ETC	IMPORTANT STUFF	NOTES/REMINDERS	APPOINTMENTS	GROCERY SHOPPING	LIVE. LOVE. SLEEP. REPEAT.
					M
					T
					W
					T
					F
					S
					S

MONDAY

TUESDAY

WEDNESDAY

THURSDAY

FRIDAY

SATURDAY-SUNDAY

Nurse Life

○ MONDAY

PRIORITIES

○ TUESDAY

○ WEDNESDAY

TO DO

○ THURSDAY

○ FRIDAY

○ SATURDAY / SUNDAY

MEALS / FOOD

MISCELLANEOUS

ME TIME - READ, WALK, RELAX, SPA, ETC	IMPORTANT STUFF	NOTES/REMINDERS	APPOINTMENTS	GROCERY SHOPPING	LIVE. LOVE. SLEEP. REPEAT.
					M
					T
					W
					T
					F
					S
					S

MONDAY

TUESDAY

WEDNESDAY

THURSDAY

FRIDAY

SATURDAY-SUNDAY

Nurse Life

○ MONDAY

PRIORITIES

○ TUESDAY

○ WEDNESDAY

TO DO

○ THURSDAY

○ FRIDAY

○ SATURDAY / SUNDAY

MEALS / FOOD

MISCELLANEOUS

ME TIME - READ, WALK, RELAX, SPA, ETC	IMPORTANT STUFF	NOTES/REMINDERS	APPOINTMENTS	GROCERY SHOPPING	LIVE. LOVE. SLEEP. REPEAT.
					M
					T
					W
					T
					F
					S
					S

MONDAY

TUESDAY

WEDNESDAY

THURSDAY

FRIDAY

SATURDAY-SUNDAY

Nurse Life

○ MONDAY

PRIORITIES

○ TUESDAY

○ WEDNESDAY

TO DO

○ THURSDAY

○ FRIDAY

○ SATURDAY / SUNDAY

MEALS / FOOD

MISCELLANEOUS

ME TIME - READ, WALK, RELAX, SPA, ETC
IMPORTANT STUFF
NOTES/REMINDERS
APPOINTMENTS
GROCERY SHOPPING
LIVE. LOVE. SLEEP. REPEAT.

						M
						T
						W
						T
						F
						S
						S

MONDAY

TUESDAY

WEDNESDAY

THURSDAY

FRIDAY

SATURDAY-SUNDAY

Nurse Life

○ MONDAY

PRIORITIES

○ TUESDAY

○ WEDNESDAY

TO DO

○ THURSDAY

○ FRIDAY

○ SATURDAY / SUNDAY

MEALS / FOOD

MISCELLANEOUS

ME TIME - READ, WALK, RELAX, SPA, ETC.	IMPORTANT STUFF	NOTES/REMINDERS	APPOINTMENTS	GROCERY SHOPPING	LIVE. LOVE. SLEEP. REPEAT.
					M
					T
					W
					T
					F
					S
					S

MONDAY

TUESDAY

WEDNESDAY

THURSDAY

FRIDAY

SATURDAY-SUNDAY

MEALS / FOOD

MISCELLANEOUS

ME TIME - READ, WALK, RELAX, SPA, ETC	IMPORTANT STUFF	NOTES/REMINDERS	APPOINTMENTS	GROCERY SHOPPING	LIVE. LOVE. SLEEP. REPEAT.
					M
					T
					W
					T
					F
					S
					S

MONDAY

TUESDAY

WEDNESDAY

THURSDAY

FRIDAY

SATURDAY-SUNDAY

Nurse Life

○ MONDAY

PRIORITIES

○ TUESDAY

○ WEDNESDAY

TO DO

○ THURSDAY

○ FRIDAY

○ SATURDAY / SUNDAY

MEALS / FOOD

MISCELLANEOUS

ME TIME - READ, WALK, RELAX, SPA, ETC	IMPORTANT STUFF	NOTES/REMINDERS	APPOINTMENTS	GROCERY SHOPPING	LIVE. LOVE. SLEEP. REPEAT.
					M
					T
					W
					T
					F
					S
					S

MONDAY

TUESDAY

WEDNESDAY

THURSDAY

FRIDAY

SATURDAY-SUNDAY

Nurse Life

○ MONDAY

PRIORITIES

○ TUESDAY

○ WEDNESDAY

TO DO

○ THURSDAY

○ FRIDAY

○ SATURDAY / SUNDAY

MEALS / FOOD

MISCELLANEOUS

ME TIME - READ, WALK, RELAX, SPA, ETC

IMPORTANT STUFF

NOTES/REMINDERS

APPOINTMENTS

GROCERY SHOPPING

LIVE. LOVE. SLEEP. REPEAT.

						M
						T
						W
						T
						F
						S
						S

MONDAY

TUESDAY

WEDNESDAY

THURSDAY

FRIDAY

SATURDAY-SUNDAY

Nurse Life

○ MONDAY

PRIORITIES

_____

○ TUESDAY

_____

○ WEDNESDAY

TO DO

_____

○ THURSDAY

_____

○ FRIDAY

_____

○ SATURDAY / SUNDAY

_____

MEALS / FOOD

MISCELLANEOUS

ME TIME - READ, WALK, RELAX, SPA, ETC	IMPORTANT STUFF	NOTES/REMINDERS	APPOINTMENTS	GROCERY SHOPPING	LIVE. LOVE. SLEEP. REPEAT.
					M
					T
					W
					T
					F
					S
					S

MONDAY

TUESDAY

WEDNESDAY

THURSDAY

FRIDAY

SATURDAY-SUNDAY

Nurse Life

○ MONDAY

PRIORITIES

○ TUESDAY

○ WEDNESDAY

TO DO

○ THURSDAY

○ FRIDAY

○ SATURDAY / SUNDAY

MEALS / FOOD

MISCELLANEOUS

ME TIME - READ, WALK, RELAX, SPA, ETC	IMPORTANT STUFF	NOTES/REMINDERS	APPOINTMENTS	GROCERY SHOPPING	LIVE. LOVE. SLEEP. REPEAT.
					M
					T
					W
					T
					F
					S
					S

MONDAY

TUESDAY

WEDNESDAY

THURSDAY

FRIDAY

SATURDAY-SUNDAY

Nurse Life

○ MONDAY

PRIORITIES

○ TUESDAY

○ WEDNESDAY

TO DO

○ THURSDAY

○ FRIDAY

○ SATURDAY / SUNDAY

MEALS / FOOD

MISCELLANEOUS

ME TIME - READ, WALK, RELAX, SPA, ETC

IMPORTANT STUFF

NOTES/REMINDERS

APPOINTMENTS

GROCERY SHOPPING

LIVE. LOVE. SLEEP. REPEAT.

M
T
W
T
F
S
S

MONDAY

TUESDAY

WEDNESDAY

THURSDAY

FRIDAY

SATURDAY-SUNDAY

Nurse Life

○ MONDAY

PRIORITIES

_____

○ TUESDAY

○ WEDNESDAY

TO DO

_____

○ THURSDAY

○ FRIDAY

○ SATURDAY / SUNDAY

MEALS / FOOD

MISCELLANEOUS

ME TIME - READ, WALK, RELAX, SPA, ETC

IMPORTANT STUFF

NOTES/REMINDERS

APPOINTMENTS

GROCERY SHOPPING

LIVE. LOVE. SLEEP. REPEAT.

M
T
W
T
F
S
S

MONDAY

TUESDAY

WEDNESDAY

THURSDAY

FRIDAY

SATURDAY-SUNDAY

Nurse Life

○ MONDAY

PRIORITIES

○ TUESDAY

○ WEDNESDAY

TO DO

○ THURSDAY

○ FRIDAY

○ SATURDAY / SUNDAY

MEALS / FOOD

MISCELLANEOUS

ME TIME - READ, WALK, RELAX, SPA, ETC	IMPORTANT STUFF	NOTES/REMINDERS	APPOINTMENTS	GROCERY SHOPPING	LIVE. LOVE. SLEEP. REPEAT.
					M
					T
					W
					T
					F
					S
					S

MONDAY

TUESDAY

WEDNESDAY

THURSDAY

FRIDAY

SATURDAY-SUNDAY

Nurse Life

○ MONDAY

PRIORITIES

○ TUESDAY

○ WEDNESDAY

TO DO

○ THURSDAY

○ FRIDAY

○ SATURDAY / SUNDAY

MEALS / FOOD

MISCELLANEOUS

ME TIME - READ, WALK, RELAX, SPA, ETC	IMPORTANT STUFF	NOTES/REMINDERS	APPOINTMENTS	GROCERY SHOPPING	LIVE. LOVE. SLEEP. REPEAT.
					M
					T
					W
					T
					F
					S
					S

MONDAY

TUESDAY

WEDNESDAY

THURSDAY

FRIDAY

SATURDAY-SUNDAY

Nurse Life

○ MONDAY

PRIORITIES

○ TUESDAY

○ WEDNESDAY

TO DO

○ THURSDAY

○ FRIDAY

○ SATURDAY / SUNDAY

MEALS / FOOD

MISCELLANEOUS

ME TIME - READ, WALK, RELAX, SPA, ETC	IMPORTANT STUFF	NOTES/REMINDERS	APPOINTMENTS	GROCERY SHOPPING	LIVE. LOVE. SLEEP. REPEAT.
					M
					T
					W
					T
					F
					S
					S

MONDAY

TUESDAY

WEDNESDAY

THURSDAY

FRIDAY

SATURDAY-SUNDAY

Nurse Life

○ MONDAY

PRIORITIES

○ TUESDAY

○ WEDNESDAY

TO DO

○ THURSDAY

○ FRIDAY

○ SATURDAY / SUNDAY

MEALS / FOOD

MISCELLANEOUS

ME TIME - READ, WALK, RELAX, SPA, ETC	IMPORTANT STUFF	NOTES/REMINDERS	APPOINTMENTS	GROCERY SHOPPING	LIVE. LOVE. SLEEP. REPEAT.
					M
					T
					W
					T
					F
					S
					S

MONDAY

TUESDAY

WEDNESDAY

THURSDAY

FRIDAY

SATURDAY-SUNDAY

Nurse Life

○ MONDAY

PRIORITIES

○ TUESDAY

○ WEDNESDAY

TO DO

○ THURSDAY

○ FRIDAY

○ SATURDAY / SUNDAY

MEALS / FOOD

MISCELLANEOUS

ME TIME - READ, WALK, RELAX, SPA, ETC	IMPORTANT STUFF	NOTES/REMINDERS	APPOINTMENTS	GROCERY SHOPPING	LIVE. LOVE. SLEEP. REPEAT.
					M
					T
					W
					T
					F
					S
					S

MONDAY

TUESDAY

WEDNESDAY

THURSDAY

FRIDAY

SATURDAY-SUNDAY

Nurse Life

○ MONDAY

PRIORITIES

○ TUESDAY

○ WEDNESDAY

TO DO

○ THURSDAY

○ FRIDAY

○ SATURDAY / SUNDAY

MEALS / FOOD

MISCELLANEOUS

ME TIME - READ, WALK, RELAX, SPA, ETC

IMPORTANT STUFF

NOTES/REMINDERS

APPOINTMENTS

GROCERY SHOPPING

LIVE. LOVE. SLEEP. REPEAT.

M
T
W
T
F
S
S

MONDAY

TUESDAY

WEDNESDAY

THURSDAY

FRIDAY

SATURDAY-SUNDAY

MEALS / FOOD

MISCELLANEOUS

ME TIME - READ, WALK, RELAX, SPA, ETC	IMPORTANT STUFF	NOTES/REMINDERS	APPOINTMENTS	GROCERY SHOPPING	LIVE. LOVE. SLEEP. REPEAT.
					M
					T
					W
					T
					F
					S
					S

MONDAY

TUESDAY

WEDNESDAY

THURSDAY

FRIDAY

SATURDAY-SUNDAY

Nurse Life

○ MONDAY

PRIORITIES

○ TUESDAY

○ WEDNESDAY

TO DO

○ THURSDAY

○ FRIDAY

○ SATURDAY / SUNDAY

MEALS / FOOD

MISCELLANEOUS

ME TIME - READ, WALK, RELAX, SPA, ETC	IMPORTANT STUFF	NOTES/REMINDERS	APPOINTMENTS	GROCERY SHOPPING	LIVE. LOVE. SLEEP. REPEAT.	
						M
						T
						W
						T
						F
						S
						S

MONDAY

TUESDAY

WEDNESDAY

THURSDAY

FRIDAY

SATURDAY-SUNDAY

Nurse Life

○ MONDAY

PRIORITIES

○ TUESDAY

○ WEDNESDAY

TO DO

○ THURSDAY

○ FRIDAY

○ SATURDAY / SUNDAY

MEALS / FOOD

MISCELLANEOUS

ME TIME - READ, WALK, RELAX, SPA, ETC	IMPORTANT STUFF	NOTES/REMINDERS	APPOINTMENTS	GROCERY SHOPPING	LIVE. LOVE. SLEEP. REPEAT.	
						M
						T
						W
						T
						F
						S
						S

MONDAY

TUESDAY

WEDNESDAY

THURSDAY

FRIDAY

SATURDAY-SUNDAY

Nurse Life

○ MONDAY

PRIORITIES

○ TUESDAY

○ WEDNESDAY

TO DO

○ THURSDAY

○ FRIDAY

○ SATURDAY / SUNDAY

MEALS / FOOD

MISCELLANEOUS

ME TIME - READ, WALK, RELAX, SPA, ETC	IMPORTANT STUFF	NOTES/REMINDERS	APPOINTMENTS	GROCERY SHOPPING	LIVE. LOVE. SLEEP. REPEAT.
					M
					T
					W
					T
					F
					S
					S

MONDAY

TUESDAY

WEDNESDAY

THURSDAY

FRIDAY

SATURDAY-SUNDAY

Nurse Life

○ MONDAY

PRIORITIES

_____

_____

_____

_____

_____

○ TUESDAY

_____

_____

_____

_____

○ WEDNESDAY

TO DO

_____

_____

○ THURSDAY

_____

_____

_____

_____

_____

○ FRIDAY

_____

_____

_____

_____

○ SATURDAY / SUNDAY

_____

_____

_____

_____

MEALS / FOOD

MISCELLANEOUS

ME TIME - READ, WALK, RELAX, SPA, ETC	IMPORTANT STUFF	NOTES/REMINDERS	APPOINTMENTS	GROCERY SHOPPING	LIVE. LOVE. SLEEP. REPEAT.
					M
					T
					W
					T
					F
					S
					S

MONDAY

TUESDAY

WEDNESDAY

THURSDAY

FRIDAY

SATURDAY-SUNDAY

Nurse Life

○ MONDAY

PRIORITIES

○ TUESDAY

○ WEDNESDAY

TO DO

○ THURSDAY

○ FRIDAY

○ SATURDAY / SUNDAY

MEALS / FOOD

MISCELLANEOUS

ME TIME - READ, WALK, RELAX, SPA, ETC	IMPORTANT STUFF	NOTES/REMINDERS	APPOINTMENTS	GROCERY SHOPPING	LIVE. LOVE. SLEEP. REPEAT.
					M
					T
					W
					T
					F
					S
					S

MONDAY

TUESDAY

WEDNESDAY

THURSDAY

FRIDAY

SATURDAY-SUNDAY

Nurse Life

○ MONDAY

○ TUESDAY

○ WEDNESDAY

○ THURSDAY

○ FRIDAY

○ SATURDAY / SUNDAY

PRIORITIES

TO DO

MEALS / FOOD

MISCELLANEOUS

ME TIME - READ, WALK, RELAX, SPA, ETC

IMPORTANT STUFF

NOTES/REMINDERS

APPOINTMENTS

GROCERY SHOPPING

LIVE. LOVE. SLEEP. REPEAT.

M
T
W
T
F
S
S

MONDAY

TUESDAY

WEDNESDAY

THURSDAY

FRIDAY

SATURDAY-SUNDAY

Nurse Life

○ MONDAY

PRIORITIES

○ TUESDAY

○ WEDNESDAY

TO DO

○ THURSDAY

○ FRIDAY

○ SATURDAY / SUNDAY

MEALS / FOOD

MISCELLANEOUS

ME TIME - READ, WALK, RELAX, SPA, ETC	IMPORTANT STUFF	NOTES/REMINDERS	APPOINTMENTS	GROCERY SHOPPING	LIVE. LOVE. SLEEP. REPEAT.
					M
					T
					W
					T
					F
					S
					S

MONDAY

TUESDAY

WEDNESDAY

THURSDAY

FRIDAY

SATURDAY-SUNDAY

Nurse Life

○ MONDAY

PRIORITIES

○ TUESDAY

○ WEDNESDAY

TO DO

○ THURSDAY

○ FRIDAY

○ SATURDAY / SUNDAY

MEALS / FOOD

MISCELLANEOUS

ME TIME - READ, WALK, RELAX, SPA, ETC

IMPORTANT STUFF

NOTES/REMINDERS

APPOINTMENTS

GROCERY SHOPPING

LIVE. LOVE. SLEEP. REPEAT.

M
T
W
T
F
S
S

MONDAY

TUESDAY

WEDNESDAY

THURSDAY

FRIDAY

SATURDAY-SUNDAY

Nurse Life

○ MONDAY

PRIORITIES

○ TUESDAY

○ WEDNESDAY

TO DO

○ THURSDAY

○ FRIDAY

○ SATURDAY / SUNDAY

Made in the USA
Lexington, KY
04 May 2019